Brain Tumor

*Discover What Your Health Practitioners
Will Never Tell You About The Tumor In
Your Brain*

Cherilyn K. Chaffin

Table of Contents

BRAIN TUMOR 1

INTRODUCTION 5

CHAPTER 1 7

   TYPES OF BRAIN CANCER 7
   FACTORS BEHIND BRAIN CANCER 9
   BRAIN CANCERS SYMPTOMS 10
      When to get Medical Care 12
   DIAGNOSING BRAIN CANCER 14

CHAPTER 2 18

   BRAIN MALIGNANCY TREATMENT 18
   BRAIN TUMOR TREATMENT OVERVIEW 18
   NEW BRAIN MALIGNANCY TREATMENTS 23
      Brain Cancer Success Rate 25
      Organizations and Counseling 26
      Home Look after Brain Cancer 28

CHAPTER 3 30

   CAUSES OF BRAIN TUMORS 30
   RISK FACTORS BRAIN TUMOR 30
   DIAGNOSIS FOR BRAIN TUMOR 30
      Treatment after treatment 30

CHAPTER 4 31

   WHEN SHOULD SOMEONE SEEK HEALTH CARE FOR BRAIN TUMOR? 31
   WHAT EXAMS AND TESTS DIAGNOSE BRAIN CANCER? 33
      What Exactly Are Treatments for Brain Cancer? 36
      Self-Care for Brain Cancer 37

CHAPTER 5 58

   WHEN LUNG MALIGNANCY SPREADS TO THE MIND 58

WHAT EXACTLY ARE THE SYMPTOMS OF LUNG MALIGNANCY SPREADING TO THE MIND? 60
HOW WILL YOU DISPLAY FOR LUNG CANCERS THAT'S SPREAD? 61
What treatments can be found? 62
Success Rates for Selected Adult Brain and SPINAL-CORD Tumors 62

CHAPTER 6 66

HOW BRAIN TUMOURS ARE GRADED 66
BRAIN CANCERS GRADES 70
EVALUATING BRAIN TUMORS 71
Type of cells or cells affected 71

CHAPTER 7 75

TUMOR MARKS AND TYPES 75
TYPES OF MAJOR BRAIN TUMORS 78
BRAIN TUMOR: LEVELS AND PROGNOSTIC FACTORS 80
Prognostic factors 81

CHAPTER 8 88

WHERE BRAIN MALIGNANCIES START AND SPREAD 88
TYPES OF BRAIN TUMORS 90
HOW BRAIN TUMOR IS TREATED 91

CHAPTER 9 93

WHAT'S GLIOBLASTOMA? 93
SYMPTOMS 94
DIAGNOSIS 95
Treatment 95
what does grade 4 astrocytoma mean? 99
Types of glioblastoma 99

ACKNOWLEDGMENTS 106

Copyright © 2022 by Cherilyn K. Chaffin

All rights reserved. No part of this publication may be reproduced, distributed, or transmitted in any form or by any means, including photocopying, recording, or other electronic or mechanical methods, without the prior written permission of the publisher, except in the case of brief quotations embodied in critical reviews and certain other non-commercial uses permitted by copyright law.

Introduction

Provides a comprehensive overview of the molecular methodologies in the neuro-oncology field.

Each year about 4,000 children and teens in the United States are diagnosed with a brain or spinal cord tumor. The illness and its treatment can have devastating effects on family, friends, schoolmates, and the larger community.

Cancers of the mind are the result of abnormal growths of cells in the mind. Brain malignancies can occur from main brain cells, the cells that form other brain components (for example, membranes, arteries), or from the development of malignancy cells that develop in other organs and which have pass on to the mind by the blood stream (metastatic or supplementary brain tumor).

Although some growths in the mind are popularly called brain tumors, not absolutely all brain tumors are cancerous. A tumor is merely scores of cells. A harmless tumor comprises cells that are not cancerous. A malignant tumor is made up of cancers cells. Malignancy is a term reserved for malignant tumors. Malignant tumors are comprised of aggressively growing, abnormal-appearing cells known as cancer cells.

This book explained medical facts, advice to ease your daily life, and tools to be a strong advocate for you, your family and friends who are suffering from brain tumor.

chapter 1

Types of Brain Cancer

- Brain tumors are abnormal growths of cells in the mind.

Although such growths are popularly called brain tumors, not absolutely all brain tumors are cancer. Tumor is a term reserved for malignant tumors.

Malignant tumors can grow and pass on aggressively, overpowering healthy cells by firmly taking their space, bloodstream, and nutrients. They are able to also pass on to distant areas of the body. Like all cells of your body, tumor cells need bloodstream and nutrition to survive.

Tumors that do not invade close by tissue or pass on to distant areas arc called benign.

Generally, a benign tumor is less serious when compared to a malignant tumor. But a harmless tumor can still cause many problems in the mind by pressing on close by tissue.

In the U.S., brain or anxious system tumors impact about 6 of each 1,000 people.

- Main Brain Cancers

The brain comprises of many types of cells.

Some brain malignancies occur when one kind of cell transforms from its normal characteristics. Once changed, the cells develop and multiply in irregular ways.

As these unusual cells grow, they turn into a mass, or tumor.

The mind tumors that result are called primary brain tumors because they originate in the mind.

The most frequent primary brain tumors are gliomas, meningiomas, pituitary adenomas, vestibular schwannomas, and primitive neuroectodermal tumors (medulloblastomas). The word glioma includes glioblastomas, astrocytomas, oligodendrogliomas, and ependymomas.

Many of these are named following the area of the brain

or the kind of brain cell that they arise.

- Metastatic Brain Cancer

Metastatic brain tumors are constructed of cancerous cells from a tumor elsewhere in the torso. The cells spread to the mind from another tumor in an activity called metastasis. That is the most typical kind of brain tumor.

Factors behind Brain Cancer

Much like tumors elsewhere in the torso, the exact reason behind most brain malignancy is unknown. Hereditary factors, various environmental poisons, radiation to the top, HIV contamination, and using tobacco have all been associated with cancers of the mind. Generally, no clear cause can be shown.

- Brain Malignancy Scans

MRI Brain Tumor Picture: Part view section through the mind of a lady. The white arrow shows a brain tumor which involves the brainstem.

- Brain Cancers MRI

MRI Brain Malignancy Picture: Cross-section (image extracted from the very best of the top down) of the brain tumor in a woman. The white arrow shows the tumor.

- Brain Tumor MRI

Brain Cancers Symptoms

Not absolutely all brain tumors cause symptoms, plus some (such as tumors of the pituitary gland) tend to be not found unless a CT check out or MRI is performed for another reason. The symptoms of brain malignancy are numerous rather than specific to brain tumors, indicating they could be triggered by a great many other ailments. The only path to find out for certain what is leading to the symptoms is to endure diagnostic screening. Symptoms can be triggered by:

- A tumor pressing on or encroaching on other areas of the mind and keeping them from working normally.

- Swelling in the mind triggered by the tumor or encircling inflammation.

The symptoms of primary and metastatic brain cancers are similar.

The next symptoms are most common:

- Headache.
- Weakness.
- Clumsiness.
- Difficulty walking.
- Seizures

Other non-specific symptoms and signals include the subsequent:

- Altered mental status -- changes in concentration, memory, attention, or alertness.
- Nausea, vomiting.
- Abnormalities in vision.

- Difficulty with speech

Progressive changes in intellectual capacity or psychological response

In lots of people, the onset of the symptoms is very gradual and could be skipped by both person with the mind tumor and the family. Sometimes, however, these symptoms show up more rapidly. Occasionally, the person functions as if they're having a heart stroke.

When to get Medical Care

Seek crisis medical help immediately if you have the following symptoms:

- Unexplained, prolonged vomiting.

- Two times vision or unexplained blurring of vision, especially on only 1 side.

- Lethargy or increased sleepiness.

- New seizures.

- New pattern or kind of headaches

Although headaches are usually a common symptom of brain cancer, they might not occur until past due in the progression of the condition. If any significant change in your headaches pattern occurs, your medical provider may claim that you go a healthcare facility.

When you have a known brain tumor, any new symptoms or relatively sudden or rapid worsening of symptoms warrants a vacation to the nearest medical center emergency department. Look for the next new symptoms:

- Seizures.

- Changes in mental position, such as excessive sleepiness, memory space problems, or failure to concentrate.

- Visible changes or other sensory problems.

- Difficulty with conversation or in expressing yourself.

- Changes in behavior or personality.

- Clumsiness or difficulty walking.

- Nausea / vomiting (especially in middle-aged or the elderly).

- Sudden onset of fever, especially after chemotherapy.

Diagnosing Brain Cancer

Results of your medical interview and physical exam will most likely suggest to your medical provider that you have trouble with the mind or brain stem.

Generally, you'll have a CT scan of the mind. This test is similar to an X-ray, but shows greater detail in three sizes. Usually, a comparison dye is injected into the bloodstream to spotlight abnormalities on the scan.

More regularly, the MRI check has been used rather than a CT check out for suspected brain tumors. It is because MRI has an increased sensitivity for discovering the existence of, or changes within, a tumor. However, most organizations still use the CT scan as the first diagnostic test.

People who have brain cancer frequently have other medical problems; therefore, regular tests may be performed. Included in these are evaluation of bloodstream, electrolytes, and liver organ function tests.

In case your mental status has been the major change, blood or urine tests may be achieved to identify drug use.

In case your scans indicate the existence of the cancerous brain tumor, you'll be described a cancer specialist, named an oncologist. If one comes in your area, you ought to be referred to an expert in brain tumors, called a neuro-oncologist.

The next phase in diagnosis is confirmation you have a cancer, usually by firmly taking and testing an example of the tumor. That is called a biopsy:

The hottest technique for finding a biopsy is surgery. The skull is opened up, usually with the purpose of removing the complete tumor, when possible. A biopsy is then extracted from the tumor.

If the doctor struggles to remove the whole tumor, a little bit of the tumor is removed.

In some instances, you'll be able to gather a biopsy without starting the skull. The precise located area of the tumor in the mind depends upon utilizing a CT or MRI scan. A little opening is then manufactured in the skull and a needle led through the opening to the tumor. The needle gathers the biopsy and it is removed. This system is named stereotaxis, or stereotactic biopsy.

The biopsy is examined under a microscope with a pathologist (a health care provider who specializes in diagnosing diseases by looking at cells and tissues).

chapter 2

Brain Malignancy Treatment

Treatment for a brain tumor differs depending on several factors: someone's age, health and wellness, and the scale, location, and kind of tumor.

You as well as your family members will have many questions about brain cancers, the treatment, part results, and the long-term perspective. Your health care and attention team is the best way to obtain this information. Please ask.

Brain Tumor Treatment Overview

Treatment of brain tumor is usually organic. Most treatment programs involve several talking to doctors.

The team of doctors includes neurosurgeons (specialists in the mind and anxious system), oncologists, radiation oncologists (doctors who practice radiation therapy), and, of course, most of your doctor. Your team could also add a dietitian, an interpersonal employee, a physical therapist, and, possibly, other specialists like a neurologist.

The procedure protocols vary widely based on the located area of the tumor, its size and type, your actual age, and any extra medical issues that you might have.

The hottest treatments are surgery, radiation therapy, and chemotherapy. Generally, several of these can be used.

- Brain Cancers Surgery

Many people who have a brain tumor undergo surgery.

The goal of surgery is to verify that the abnormality seen during testing is definitely a tumor and also to take away the tumor. If the tumor can't be removed, the cosmetic surgeon will take an example of the tumor to recognize its type.

In some instances, mostly in benign tumors, symptoms can be completely cured by surgery of the tumor. The neurosurgeon will try to remove all the tumor when possible.

You might undergo several treatments and procedures before surgery. For instance:

You might be given a steroid medication, such as dexamethasone (Decadron), to alleviate swelling.

You might be treated with an anticonvulsant medication to alleviate or prevent seizures.

When you have excess cerebrospinal liquid collecting around the mind, a thin, plastic material pipe called a shunt may be positioned to drain the liquid. One end of the shunt is positioned in the cavity where liquid gathers; the other end is threaded under your skin layer to a different area of the body. The liquid drains from the mind to a niche site that the liquid can be easily removed.

- Rays Therapy for Brain Cancer

Rays therapy (also known as radiotherapy) is the utilization of high-energy rays to kills tumor cells, thereby stopping them from growing and multiplying.

Radiation therapy can be utilized for individuals who cannot undergo surgery. In other instances, it is utilized after surgery to destroy any tumor cells that may stay.

Rays therapy is an area therapy. Which means that it impacts only cells in its route. It typically will not damage cells elsewhere in the torso or even somewhere else in the mind.

Radiation can get in the next ways:

- External radiation runs on the high-energy beam of radiation directed at the tumor. The beam moves through your skin, the skull, healthy brain tissue, and other tissue to access the tumor. The treatments are usually given five times weekly for a degree of time. Each treatment requires just a few minutes.

- Internal or implant radiation runs on the small radioactive capsule that is positioned inside the tumor itself. Rays emitted from the capsule destroys the tumor. The radioactivity of the capsule reduces a bit each day and it is carefully determined to perform out when the perfect dosage has been given. You will need to stay the hospital for a number of days while getting this treatment.

- Stereotactic radiosurgery may also be called a "knifeless" medical technique, though it generally does not involve surgery. It destroys a brain tumor without starting the skull. A CT or MRI check out is utilized to pinpoint the precise located area of the tumor in the mind. An individual large dosage of high-energy rays beams are trained on the tumor from different perspectives. Rays destroys the tumor. Stereotactic radiosurgery has fewer problems than open up surgery and a shorter recovery time.

- Chemotherapy for Brain Cancer

Chemotherapy is the utilization of powerful drugs to get rid of tumor cells.

A single medication or a mixture of drugs can be utilized.

The drugs receive orally or via an IV collection. Some medications receive through the shunt devote spot to drain extra fluid from the mind.

Chemotherapy is usually given in cycles. A routine consists of a brief period of rigorous treatment accompanied by an interval of rest and recovery. Each routine lasts a couple weeks.

Most regimens were created so that two to four cycles are completed. There is certainly a break in the procedure to observe how your tumor has been taken care of immediately after therapy.

The side ramifications of chemotherapy are popular. They might be very hard to tolerate for a lot of time. They could include nausea and throwing up, mouth sores, lack of appetite, lack of hair, amongst others. A few of these side results can be relieved or improved by medication.

New Brain Malignancy Treatments

New therapies for tumor are being developed on a regular

basis. Whenever a therapy shows guarantee, it is analyzed in a laboratory and improved whenever you can. It really is then examined in clinical tests involving people who have cancer.

Through brain cancer medical trials, researchers test the consequences of new medications on several volunteers with brain cancer. Patients with brain malignancy may be hesitant to be a part of clinical studies for concern with getting no treatment whatsoever for his or her brain cancer.

Clinical trials are for sale to practically every kind of cancer.

The benefit of clinical trials is that they provide new therapies which may be far better than existing therapies or have fewer side effects.

The disadvantage is that the treatment is not which can work or might not work in everyone.

Many people who have cancer meet the criteria for participation in scientific trials.

For more information, ask your oncologist. A summary of clinical tests is offered by the website of the Country wide Cancer Institute.

Once a brain tumor is diagnosed, you should be careful to keep all visits with consultants as well as your primary doctor. People who have brain cancers often are in increased risk for more medical problems and, possibly, recurrence of malignancy or a worsening of their symptoms.

Brain Cancer Success Rate

Survival rates in brain tumor vary widely. The major factors that impact survival are the kind of cancers, its location, whether it could be surgically removed or low in size, your actual age, and other medical problems.

In general, more youthful patients have a much better prognosis.

Brain malignancy that has pass on (or metastasized) from

someplace else in the torso is the most typical type. Success rates rely on the initial malignancy and other factors.

Treatment for some types of brain cancers is available and can often offer you a better potential for survival. Discuss treatment plans and best-estimated prognosis with your tumor team.

Organizations and Counseling

Living with cancers presents many new issues, both for you and for your friends and relations.

You will likely have many worries about how exactly the cancer will affect you as well as your ability to "live a standard life;" that is, to look after your loved ones and home, to carry your job, and also to carrying on the friendships and activities you love.

Many people feel stressed and depressed. Some individuals feel upset and resentful; others feel helpless and defeated.

For many people with cancer, discussing their emotions and concerns helps.

Friends and family can be quite supportive. They might be hesitant to provide support until they observe how you are coping. Don't await them to take it up. If you wish to discuss concerns, tell them.

Some individuals don't want to "burden" themselves, or prefer discussing their concerns with a far more natural professional. A interpersonal employee, counselor, or person in the clergy may be helpful if you would like to discuss emotions and concerns about having malignancy. Your oncologist can recommend someone.

Many people who have cancer are helped profoundly by speaking with others who have cancer. Posting concerns with other people who have experienced the same experience can be amazingly reassuring. Organizations of individuals with tumor may be accessible through the infirmary what your location is getting treatment. The American Cancers Society also offers information about organizations all around the U.S.

Home Look after Brain Cancer

When fighting brain cancers, your wellbeing care team will discuss information regarding home care with your household members.

Home treatment usually includes supportive steps, depending on your symptoms and person needs.

For instance, if you have trouble walking, physical and occupational therapists will help you improve motion and use equipment to assist in day to day activities.

A talk therapist can help with problems related to speaking and swallowing. Home health aides are specially trained to assist with personal care jobs such as bathing, dressing, and eating.

Home treatment can likewise incorporate nurses to provide medicines, provide wound treatment, and monitor aspect effects.

If the prognosis is poor, it is suitable to go over options including hospice care, advance directives to doctors, and procedures for a full time income will.

Home hospice treatment is a means of providing pain and symptom alleviation, as well as psychological and religious support for the individual and the family, at home rather than in a healthcare facility. It entails a multidisciplinary approach that can include a health care provider or other doctor, nurses, a pharmacist, aides, a sociable worker, a religious caregiver, and counselors.

Progress directives are legal documents offering a way to express your desires for treatment as well as your choice on the individual you want to make decisions in your stead if you aren't able to do this. Types of progress directives add a living will and durable power of lawyer for healthcare. For instance, a person with advanced brain malignancy may not desire to be placed on a ventilator (deep breathing machine) if she or he stops respiration. You have to make these decisions for yourself so long as you are psychologically competent.

chapter 3

chapter 4

When Should Someone Seek Health Care for Brain Tumor?

Seek treatment from physician immediately, probably emergently, if a person develops the following symptoms:

- Unexplained, continual vomiting.

- Increase vision or unexplained blurring of vision, especially on only 1 side.

- Lethargy or increased sleepiness.

- New seizures.

- New pattern or kind of headaches, especially morning hours headaches

Although headaches are usually a common symptom of brain cancer, they might not occur until past due in the progression of the condition. If any significant change in someone's headache design occurs rapidly, healthcare professionals may claim that she or he go the crisis department. If one has a known brain tumor, any new symptoms or relatively unexpected or quick worsening of symptoms also warrants a vacation to the nearest medical center emergency department. Look for the next new symptoms:

- Seizures.

- Changes in mental position, such as excessive sleepiness, memory space problems, or lack of ability to concentrate.

- Visible changes or other sensory problems.

- Difficulty with conversation or in expressing oneself.

- Changes in behavior or personality.

- Clumsiness or difficulty walking.

- Nausea / vomiting (especially in middle-aged or the elderly).

- Sudden onset of fever, particularly if the individual

is getting chemotherapy treatments.

What Exams and Tests Diagnose Brain Cancer?

If findings of the health background and physical exam suggest to medical care professional a person having issues in the mind or brain stem, additional assessments may be achieved.

Many people will have a CT scan of the mind, especially if the individual sometimes appears emergently.

This test is similar to an X-ray but shows greater detail in three dimensions.

Usually, a dye, known as a contrast material, is injected in to the bloodstream to highlight abnormalities on the scan.

People who have brain cancer frequently have other medical problems; therefore, regular laboratory checks may be performed.

Included in these are analysis of bloodstream,

electrolytes, liver organ function testing, and a bloodstream coagulation (clotting) profile.

If the individual has mental-status change as the primary sign, blood or urine tests may be achieved to eliminate drug use as a reason behind such symptoms.

The typical way of evaluating the type and extent of the brain tumor can be an MRI scan (remember that some hospitals don't have MRI scanners).

It is because MRI has an increased sensitivity for discovering the existence and characteristics of the tumor. Specifically, the partnership of the tumor to the encompassing brain, the mind coverings, cerebrospinal liquid areas, and vascular constructions is assessed to create a provisional analysis of the type of the tumor.

Presently, however, many institutions that do have MRI scanners still use the CT scan as a screening test for tumors.

If CT or MRI scans indicate the existence of the brain

tumor, the individual will be described brain surgery (a neurosurgeon). If one comes in the area, the individual can also be known an expert in rays therapy called a rays oncologist, and a medical oncologist if indeed they focus on the chemotherapeutic treatment of brain tumors (a medical or neuro-oncologist).

The next phase in diagnosis is confirmation that the individual has cancer in the mind. A scan can be viewed as to be highly dubious, or even highly more likely to demonstrate a brain tumor, but verification requires a cells diagnosis whenever you can. A small test of the tumor (a biopsy) is taken up to identify the kind of tumor and the standard of the tumor.

The hottest technique for finding a biopsy is a medical procedure called a craniotomy. The skull is opened up, usually with the purpose of removing the complete tumor when possible. A biopsy is then extracted from the tumor.

If the physician struggles to remove the whole tumor, a

little bit of the tumor is removed.

In some instances, you'll be able to gather a biopsy without starting the skull. The precise located area of the tumor in the mind is set stereotactically, that is, by using CT or MRI scans as the mind is kept still in a framework. A small gap is then manufactured in the skull and a needle led through the opening to the tumor. The needle gathers the biopsy and it is removed. This system is named stereotaxis, or stereotactic biopsy. This technique will not treat the tumor and is normally reserved for situations where the tumor is either inaccessible or is regarded as sensitive to rays therapy (such as CNS lymphoma or pineal germ cell tumor) and surgery is not essential to properly treat the individual.

The biopsy is examined under a microscope with a pathologist (your physician who specializes in diagnosing diseases by looking at cells and tissues) and usually assigned a NCI grade.

What Exactly Are Treatments for Brain Cancer?

Treatment for brain cancers should be individualized for every patient. Treatment programs derive from the patient's age group and health and wellness position as well as the scale, location, type, and grade of the tumor. Generally of brain malignancy, surgery, rays, and chemotherapy are the primary types of treatment. Often, several treatment type can be used. The procedure types are further explained below.

The individual, family, and friends will have many questions about the tumor, the procedure, how treatment will affect the individual, and the individuals long-term outlook (prognosis). Users of the individuals healthcare team will be the best way to obtain this information. Please inquire further any questions.

Self-Care for Brain Cancer

The person's doctor and the physician team responsible for their case should discuss information regarding home care with both patient and family.

Home treatment usually includes supportive actions needed based on the patient's symptoms. For instance, walkers may get for those patients who've gait or small balance problems.

If one has mental-status changes, a care plan should be directed to the patient's individual needs. For instance, a caregiver may be designated to manage the patient's daily medications.

If the patient's prognosis is poor, it is suitable to go over options of hospice care and advance directives with the doctors.

Home hospice treatment is a means of providing pain and symptom alleviation, as well as emotional and religious support for the individual and the family, at home rather than in a healthcare facility. It requires a multidisciplinary approach that can include your physician or other caution supplier, nurses, a pharmacist, aides, a cultural worker, a religious caregiver, and counselors.

Progress directives and living wills are legal documents that explain specifically which treatments should be given and which should be withheld. For instance, a person with advanced brain tumor may not desire to be placed on a ventilator (deep breathing machine) if she or he stops respiration. Patients hate to make these decisions for themselves so long as they stay mentally competent. They could also desire to designate you to definitely make such decisions to them as long as they become struggling to achieve this later. Such a record is named a durable power of lawyer for healthcare decisions. Directives should be accessible to healthcare personnel, particularly when any emergent change in the individuals condition occurs, normally a person's treatment directives might not be done.

Home cures claiming remedies for brain malignancy are available on the web; they range between taking folic acidity supplements to taking antioxidants and natural substances. There is certainly little if any data to aid these statements; people are urged to go over these treatments, prior to trying them, using their doctors.

What Are MEDICAL PROCEDURES Programs for Brain Cancer?

The procedure protocols vary widely based on the located area of the tumor, its size, grade, and type, the patient's age, and any extra medical issues that the individual may have.

The hottest treatments are surgery, radiation therapy, and chemotherapy. As stated in some instances, several of the treatment types can be used.

A lot of people with a brain tumor undergo surgery. (Craniotomy is the word used to make reference to the surgical starting of the skull.)

The purposes of surgery are to verify that the abnormality seen on the mind scan is definitely a tumor, to assign a grade to the tumor, and also to take away the tumor. If the tumor can't be removed completely, the doctor will at least have a test of the tumor to recognize its type and grade.

In some instances, mostly in benign tumors, the condition can be completely cured by surgery of the tumor. A neurosurgeon will try to take away the tumor when possible.

Patients may undergo several treatments and methods before surgery.

They might be given a steroid medication, such as dexamethasone (Decadron), to alleviate swelling.

They might be treated with an anticonvulsant medication, such as levetiracetam (Keppra), phenytoin (Dilantin), or carbamazepine (Tegretol), to alleviate or prevent seizures.

Summary of Surgery for Resection of Brain Tumor

The objective of surgery for tumors is to eliminate as a lot of the tumor as is safely possible with the minimal possible loss in brain function. The top most patients undergo this process under general anesthesia. Some surgeries are done awake or under light sedation for the intended purpose of mapping vocabulary function. For surgery done under general anesthesia, an endotracheal pipe is positioned, while for those done awake, a laryngeal face mask airway (or no airway) is positioned and the individual is deeply sedated. The top is appropriately situated utilizing a clamp system that keeps the skull motionless. An image-guided navigation system is often used to help determine the complete located area of the incision. The head is prepped, following the locks is clipped, the prepared incision collection is infiltrated with local anesthesia, and the head is then incised and forced apart to expose the skull bone. Some of the skull is briefly slice away and the liner tissues of the mind are opened. If it's essential to determine whether brain function is jeopardized, the individual is awakened from sedation to be able to react as mapping methods are completed.

In any case, tumor resection is then completed. Some of the tumor is usually delivered to a pathologist for evaluation. The surgeon could also opt to place biodegradable polymer wafers that deliver chemotherapy drugs (Gliadel wafers) in to the tumor cavity. After the tumor resection is complete, the membranes encircling the mind are shut and the skull is shut, often by using titanium plates and screws that help keep it rigidly in its desired position. The head is shut; some cosmetic surgeons use drains positioned under the head for a day or two after surgery to reduce the build up of bloodstream or fluid.

Stereotactic radiosurgery is a more recent "knifeless" technique that destroys a brain tumor without starting the skull. CT or MRI scan is utilized to pinpoint the precise located area of the tumor in the mind. High-energy rays beams are trained on the tumor from different sides. Rays destroys the tumor. Equipment i did so radiosurgery varies in its rays source; a gamma blade uses concentrated gamma rays, and a linear accelerator uses photons, while heavy-charged particle radiosurgery runs on the proton beam.

The benefits of knifeless procedures are they have fewer problems and the recovery time is a lot shorter. Disadvantages are the lack of cells open to send to a pathologist for medical diagnosis and brain bloating that may appear after the rays therapy.

When there is excess cerebrospinal liquid buildup due to a blockage of liquid passageways by the tumor, a thin plastic material pipe called a shunt may be positioned to drain the liquid. One end of the shunt is positioned in the cavity where liquid gathers, and the other is threaded under your skin to a different area of the body. The liquid drains from the mind to a niche site that the liquid can be easily removed.

Inoperable Brain Tumors

Inoperable tumors are the ones that are positioned in an inaccessible put in place the mind that brain surgeons cannot reach. On the other hand, although they might be in a position to reach the tumor, to eliminate it, the doctors may need to eliminate or harm a lot nearby brain tissues so the surgery may harm the patient just as much as the tumor. Inoperable tumors can be of any type or size. Why is a tumor inoperable is if a doctor is confident they can gain access to the tumor without disrupting other significant brain tissue such as those essential for essential body functions (for example, talk or motion). Other tumors are considered inoperable when these are so penetrated by arteries that removal of the tumor and its own vascular system will probably severely harm or cause loss of life in the individual. The cosmetic surgeon determines if a patient's brain tumor is inoperable, so that it is advisable to get another opinion from another physician as another brain doctor may consider the tumor to be "operable." Doctors sometimes use whole-brain rays therapy (WBRT) to take care of inoperable brain tumors over weeks.

Rays, Chemotherapy, and Clinical Tests for Brain Cancer

Rays therapy (also known as radiotherapy) is the utilization of high-energy rays to wipe out tumor cells and stop them from growing and multiplying.

Radiation therapy may also be used for individuals who cannot undergo surgery. In other instances, it can be used after surgery to eliminate any tumor cells that may stay. Tomotherapy can be utilized (modulated rays therapy aided by CT checking).

Rays therapy is an area therapy. Which means that it impacts only cells in its route. It generally does not damage cells elsewhere in the torso or even somewhere else in the mind.

Rays can be administered in either of two ways.

External radiation runs on the high-energy beam of radiation directed at the tumor. The beam moves through your skin, the skull, healthy brain tissue, and other cells to access the tumor. The treatments are usually given five times a week for approximately 4-6 weeks. Each treatment will take just a few minutes. The gamma blade and cyber blade are two conditions that explain methods that use exterior radiation to destroy malignancy cells in the mind.

Internal or implant radiation runs on the small radioactive capsule that is positioned inside the tumor itself. Rays emitted from the capsule destroys the tumor. The radioactivity of the capsule reduces a bit each day; the quantity of radioactivity of the capsule is carefully computed to perform out when the perfect dose has been given. One must stay in a healthcare facility for several times while getting this treatment.

Chemotherapy is the utilization of powerful drugs to get rid of tumor cells.

A single medication or a mixture can be utilized.

Old drugs used to take care of brain cancers include BCNU and CCNU, procarbazine, and vincristine. Some receive by mouth, while some may get into the blood stream (IV).

Two drugs, temozolomide (Temodar) and bevacizumab (Avastin), are approved for the treating malignant gliomas. They may be more effective and also have fewer undesireable effects in comparison to old drugs. Temozolomide has another benefit for the reason that it is given orally, eliminating the necessity for intravenous lines and medical center or clinic remains for chemotherapy.

Chemotherapy is usually given in cycles. A routine consists of a brief period of extensive treatment accompanied by an interval of rest and recovery. Each routine lasts a couple weeks.

Most regimens were created so that two to four cycles are completed. There is certainly a break in the procedure, and scans are done to observe how the tumor has taken care of immediately therapy.

The side ramifications of chemotherapy are popular and

are today less complicated to tolerate. They include nausea and throwing up, mouth sores, lack of appetite, lack of hair, and many more. A few of these side results can be relieved or improved by medication.

New therapies (for example, use of nanotechnology to provide drugs to tumor cells) for cancers are being developed on a regular basis. Whenever a research therapy shows guarantee, it is examined in laboratories and improved whenever you can. It really is then examined on people who have cancer; these checks are called scientific trials.

Clinical trials are for sale to practically every kind of cancer.

The benefit of clinical trials is that they provide new therapies which may be far better than existing therapies or have fewer side effects.

The disadvantage is that the treatment is not which can work or can not work in everyone.

Many people who have cancer meet the criteria for

participation in medical trials.

For more information, ask a healthcare professional. A summary of scientific trials is offered by the website of the Country wide Cancer Institute.

There are numerous "holistic" and other treatments for brain tumors cited in Web sites, health magazines, and other publications (for example, Transfer Factor, Cellect, Vitalzym). Many of these have no medical data to bolster their promises and, when going to these sites, visitors are urged to learn the small print because so many say the merchandise(s) aren't designed to treat specific diseases. Patients should discuss such substances using their doctors before buying and using these things. Some are outlined by the FDA as health supplements and warn they have not been became effective or safe.

What Are UNWANTED EFFECTS of Brain Cancer Treatments?

Treatment plans make an effort to limit or reduce aspect results associated with brain malignancy treatment. However, most patients will experience some part effects;

some aspect results can be severe. Individuals who go through brain tumor treatment should enquire about the potential part results and help decide if the suggested treatment(s) will be well worth the huge benefits and how to proceed if aspect effects appear.

Unwanted effects of chemotherapy can include nausea, vomiting, hair thinning, and weakness. The disease fighting capability is usually suppressed, making the individual more vulnerable to attacks. Other body organ systems like the kidneys or reproductive organs may be broken. Although these part effects usually decrease as treatment ends, some might not, particularly if other body organ systems are broken.

Rays therapy has aspect results much like those in the above list for chemotherapy, but because some body organ systems do not get a direct rays dose, the medial side results can be significantly less than those of chemotherapy. However, skin surface damage (reddish or darkened) and pores and skin sensitivity might occur. Hair thinning can also happen, especially in areas where in fact the rays enters your body; some hair thinning is permanent.

Surgery can cause both short-term and long term changes. Unwanted effects such as brain bloating, harm to normal cells, mental-status changes, muscle weakness, or changes in virtually any brain-controlled function might occur. Although such part effects usually drop as time passes, some could become permanent.

Patients and brain cancers associates should carefully consider aspect effects; often a few of them can be reduced by treatment and might not be everlasting. Brain malignancy patients who are applicants for treatment should comprehend that without surgery, chemotherapy, or rays therapy (or mixtures of these) the prognosis or view for some patients is poor.

Brain Cancers Follow-up

Once a brain tumor is diagnosed, the individual must be careful to keep all sessions with consultants and the principal doctor. In general, people who have brain cancer are in increased risk for extra medical problems and, possibly, reoccurrence or worsening of their symptoms. Survivor treatment plans summarizing both treatments an individual has received and suggestions for follow-up and indicator management should be requested of the dealing with doctors.

After treatment, patients will be returning for follow-up visits using their cancer associates. A routine of follow-up checkups and exams will be suggested. The goal of this follow-up is to ensure that any recurrence of tumor or any long-term after-effect of the procedure is identified quickly such that it can be treated immediately.

HOW DO People Prevent Brain Malignancy?

In general, there is absolutely no known way to avoid brain malignancies. However, early analysis and treatment of tumors that have a tendency to metastasize to the mind may decrease the threat of metastatic brain tumors. Avoiding or reducing connection with radiation (especially to the top) and avoiding toxic chemicals from the oil and rubber industry, embalming chemicals, and other environmental toxins can help prevent brain cancers. Avoiding HIV infection is also suggested.

The favorite press plus some internet sites claim that avoiding mobile phone use and utilizing a macrobiotic diet can help avoid brain cancer. Presently, there is absolutely no good proof for these statements. In Dec 2010, a big study around 59,000 cellular phone users, with use times varying over five to a decade, claims that no substantial change in brain cancer incidence could be within them. Investigators claim that "high usage" of mobile phones over very long time periods is yet to be investigated. The National Cancer Institute in 2016 published findings from several studies that summarize findings; most do not show any relation between mobile phone use and cancer. However, for individuals who want to reduce any radiation dose from mobile phones, the reader can seek advice from the net for a summary of phones that produce the best and lowest radiation levels.

WHAT'S the Prognosis for Brain Tumor? What Is the life span Expectancy for Someone With Brain Cancers?

Readers Remarks 17 Talk about Your Story

The major factor(s) that influence brain cancer survival relates to the next: the kind of cancer, its location, whether it could be surgically removed or reduced, and this and general health status of the individual.

The long-term survival rate (life span higher than five years) for individuals with primary brain cancer varies. In situations of intense or high-grade brain malignancies, it is from significantly less than 10% to about 32%, despite intense surgery, rays, and chemotherapy treatments.

Treatments do prolong survival on the short-term and, perhaps moreover, improve standard of living for quite a while, although this time around period may differ greatly.

Rays after surgery may increase a patient's expected success when compared with not getting it in any way. Chemotherapy can further lengthen life for a few patients when given during and/or after rays therapy.

Individuals who have continuing seizures that are difficult to regulate despite having medications generally do poorly over the next six months.

Despite seemingly dismal likelihood of long-term survival, these it's likely that clearly higher with treatment than without. Treatment plans and best-estimated prognosis should be discussed with the patient's cancer team.

Brain Cancer ORGANIZATIONS, Information, and Counseling

Living with cancers presents many new issues for the individual and their relatives and buddies.

Patients have many concerns about how exactly the malignancy will impact them and their capability to "live a standard life," that is, to look after family and home, to carry a job, and also to continue friendships and activities.

Many people feel stressed and depressed. Some individuals feel furious and resentful; others feel helpless and defeated.

For many people with cancer, discussing their emotions

and concerns helps.

Relatives and buddies members can be quite supportive. They might be hesitant to provide support until they observe how the individual is dealing with the condition. If patients want to discuss their concerns, the individual should be motivated to take action with their relatives and buddies.

Some individuals don't want to "burden" themselves or they prefer discussing their concerns with a far more natural professional. A social worker, counselor, or person in the clergy are a good idea if an individual wants to go over their feelings and concerns about having cancer. The patient's oncologist can recommend someone. For patients with terminal cancer, hospice can help both patient and family members in this difficult time.

Many people who have cancer are helped profoundly by speaking with others who have cancer. Writing concerns with other people who have experienced a similar thing can be incredibly reassuring. Organizations of individuals with tumor may be accessible through the infirmary what your location is getting your treatment. The American Malignancy Society also offers information about organizations all around the United States.

chapter 5

When Lung Malignancy Spreads to the mind

When cancer begins in a single place within you and spreads to some other, it's called metastasis. When lung malignancy metastasizes to the mind, it means the principal lung cancer has generated a secondary malignancy in the mind.

About 20 to 40 percent Trusted Way to obtain adults with non-small cell lung cancer continue to build up brain metastases sooner or later throughout their illness. The most typical metastatic sites are:

- adrenal gland.

- brain and nervous system.

- Bones.

- Liver.

- other lung or the respiratory system

So how exactly does lung tumor spread to the mind?

You will find 2 different types of lung cancer:

- small cell lung cancer, that are about 10 to 15 percent of most lung cancers.

- non-small cell lung cancer, that are about 80 to 85 percent of most lung cancers.

- Lung malignancies most typically pass on to other areas of your body through the lymph vessels and arteries.

While it's easier for lung cancer to pass on through the lymph vessels, it generally takes much longer before secondary metastatic cancer takes hold. With arteries, it's usually harder for the cancers to get into. However, once it can, it spreads relatively quickly.

In most cases, metastasis through the blood cells is worse for a while, and metastasis through lymph cells is worse in the long run.

What exactly are the symptoms of lung malignancy spreading to the mind?

If you're identified as having lung tumor, it's especially important to focus on symptoms of brain metastasis, including:

- decreases in memory space, attention, and reasoning.
- head aches caused by inflammation in the mind.
- Weakness.
- nausea and vomiting.
- Unsteadiness.
- difficulty speaking.
- Numbness.
- tingling sensations.
- seizures

When you have these symptoms, statement these to your

physician immediately.

How will you display for lung cancers that's spread?

To display screen for metastatic brain malignancy, doctors commonly use radiology assessments such as:

- MRI.
- CT scan

Occasionally, a health care provider might take a biopsy to see whether there's brain cancer present.

What's the life span expectancy for lung tumor that's pass on to the mind?

While sex, ethnicity, and age make a difference survival, the life span expectancy after an analysis of brain metastases from lung malignancy is normally poor. With no treatment, the average success rate is under 6 months Trusted Source. With treatment, that quantity can increase somewhat.

Usually those who develop brain metastases further away from diagnosis have a somewhat higher survival rate than those whose lung cancer metastasizes to the mind previously. The difference, however, is usually small.

What treatments can be found?

With regards to treatment of lung cancer brain metastases, the available choices depend on a number of different factors, such as:

- the sort of primary cancer that was diagnosed.
- the quantity, size, and location of brain tumors.
- the genetic behavior of the cancer cells.
- age group and health.
- other attempted treatments

Success Rates for Selected Adult Brain and SPINAL-CORD Tumors

Survival rates are ways to get an over-all notion of the perspective (prognosis) for individuals with a certain kind of tumor. They let you know what portion of individuals with the same kind of tumor remain alive a degree of time (usually 5 years) once they were diagnosed. They can't let you know how long you will live, however they may help offer you a much better understanding about how exactly likely it is that your treatment will achieve success.

Exactly what is a 5-year success rate?

The 5-year survival rate is the percentage of individuals who live at least 5 years after being diagnosed. For instance, a 5-12 months success rate of 70% means an approximated 70 out of 100 individuals who have that kind of tumor remain alive 5 years after being diagnosed. Remember, however, that lots of the people live a lot longer than 5 years.

Comparative survival rates (like the numbers below) are a far more accurate way to estimate the result of cancer on survival. These rates compare people who have cancer to the people in the entire population. For instance, if the

5-yr relative success rate for a particular kind of tumor is 70%, it could mean that individuals who've that kind of tumor are, normally, about 70% as likely as people who don't have that tumor to live for at least 5 years after being diagnosed.

But remember, the 5-season relative success rates are estimations - your outlook may differ based on lots of factors specific for you.

Survival rates don't show the complete story

Survival rates tend to be based on earlier outcomes of good sized quantities of individuals who had the condition, however they can't predict exactly what will happen in virtually any particular person's case. There are a few limitations to keep in mind:

These numbers are being among the most current available. But to get 5-calendar year survival rates, doctors have to check out people who have been treated at least 5 years back. As treatments are enhancing over time, folks who are now being identified as having brain or spinal-cord tumors may have a much better view than these figures show.

The outlook for individuals with brain or spinal-cord tumors varies by the kind of tumor and the person's age. But a great many other factors can also impact a person's perspective, such as how old they are and general health, where in fact the tumor is situated, and exactly how well the tumor responds to treatment. The view for every person is specific with their circumstances.

Your physician can let you know how these figures may connect with you, as they're familiar with your position.

chapter 6

How brain tumours are graded

Brain tumours are graded 1-4 according with their behaviour, like the speed of which they may be growing, and exactly how likely these are to pass on into the areas of the mind. As time passes, some brain tumour's behavior can transform and the tumour could become, or keep coming back as, an increased grade tumour.

Each year in the united kingdom, approximately 4,300 people are identified as having low grade, sluggish growing brain tumours and 5,000 with high grade fast growing brain tumours. Mixed, this represents significantly less than 2 from every 10,000 people in the united kingdom.

Brain tumours are graded from 1 - 4 depending about how they will probably behave.

Grade 1 and 2 tumours (low grade)

Grade 3 and 4 tumours (high grade)

Confirming the diagnosis of the various marks of brain tumours is performed, where possible, by analysing cells from the tumour, used throughout a biopsy or during surgery. A neuropathologist examines the cells in the lab, looking for particular cell patterns that are grade of the various types and grade of brain tumour.

Newly diagnosed?

Our free Brain Tumour Information Pack was created to help you, feeling confident when talking about treatment and care and attention with your medical team.

Order your FREE pack

How come the grade are important?

Accurate diagnosis is important as it allows your medical team to offer information about how exactly the tumour could behave in the foreseeable future, and to recommend treatment plans. This could add a clinical trial.

Sometimes confirming the grade can be difficult as some low grade and high grade tumours can look virtually identical.

Low grade tumours

Low grade brain tumours are:

- slow growing.

- relatively contained with well-defined edges.

- unlikely to pass on to other areas of the mind.

- have less chance coming back (if indeed they can be completely removed).

Grade 1 and 2 tumours are low grade, slow growing, relatively contained and unlikely to pass on to other areas of the mind. Additionally there is less potential for them returning if indeed they can be completely removed. They are occasionally still known as 'harmless'.

The word 'benign' is less used nowadays as this is deceptive. These low grade brain tumours can be serious.

It is because the tumour can cause harm by pressing on and damaging close by regions of the mind, because of the limited space capacity of the skull. They are able to also impede the flow of the cerebrospinal fluid (CSF) that nourishes and protects the mind, leading to a build-up of strain on the brain.

High grade tumours

High grade brain tumours are:

- fast growing.
- can be known as 'malignant' or 'cancerous' growths.
- much more likely to pass on to other areas of the mind.
- may come back again, even if intensively treated.

Grade 3 and 4 tumours are high grade, fast growing and can be known as 'malignant' or 'cancerous' growths.

They will spread to other areas of the mind (and, rarely, the spinal-cord) and could keep coming back, even if intensively treated. They can not usually be treated by surgery only, but often require other treatments, such as radiotherapy and/or chemotherapy.

'Mixed grade' tumours

Some tumours include a combination of cells with different levels. The tumour is graded based on the highest grade of cell it includes, even if nearly all it is low grade.

Brain cancers grades

The staging process assesses the spread of cancer beyond the initial site. Brain malignancy will not behave just as other malignancies. Tumors may migrate within the mind, but it's very uncommon for main brain tumors to pass on outside of the mind, or from the central anxious system (CNS).

As a result, brain cancer is usually graded rather than staged. The mind tumor grading system features four unique grades and your caution team with a knowledge of the way the tumor develops. This technique helps doctors match brain tumor treatments to specific needs.

Evaluating brain tumors

To look for the development of tumors in the mind, doctors concentrate on the characteristics of the tumor and its own effect on features. The primary factors used to evaluate brain tumors include:

- Size and location

Type of cells or cells affected

- Resectability (the chance that part or all the tumor can be removed by surgery).
- The spread of the cancer within the mind or spinal-cord.

- The probability the cancer has spread beyond the mind or CNS.

- An entire assessment will also element in age and brain cancers symptoms that are restricting basic functions, such as conversation, hearing or motion.

- Brain malignancy grading is a lot unique of staging other malignancies in the torso. Malignancies in the lung, digestive tract and breasts are staged predicated on their location in the torso, size, lymph node participation and possible pass on.

- Tumors in the mind are graded centered on how intense the tumor cells show up under a microscope.

The grade and resectability of the tumor can help guide treatment decisions. Surgery depends upon the tumor's convenience (location), size, degree (pass on within the mind) and the patient's general health (including health background).

Grade I (grade 1 brain tumor): The tumor grows slowly and rarely spreads into close by tissues. It might be possible to totally take away the tumor with surgery.

Grade II (grade 2 brain cancers): The tumor grows slowly but may pass on into nearby cells or recur.

Grade III (grade 3 brain malignancy): The tumor grows quickly, will probably spread into close by tissue, and the tumor cells look completely different from normal cells.

Grade IV (grade 4 brain tumor): The tumor grows and spreads rapidly, and the tumor cells do not appear to be normal cells.

Metastatic brain tumors: Supplementary, or metastatic, brain tumors, that have distributed to the mind from another location in the torso, are a lot more common than major brain tumors. These tumors are also becoming more and more prevalent as individuals do better with cancers treatment and live much longer, giving the initial cancer the chance to pass on to the mind.

Some malignancies that commonly pass on to the mind are lung, breasts, digestive tract, kidney, melanoma, thyroid and uterine. Lung malignancy is the most typical form of metastatic brain malignancy. Actually, lung tumor staging often entails a brain check out.

Metastatic brain cancers is going to be assessed through the Tumor, Node, Metastasized (pass on) staging system (TNM). Sometimes, folks are identified as having metastatic brain or vertebral tumor before they realize they have another, principal cancer.

chapter 7

Tumor Marks and Types

When most normal cells get old or get damaged, they die, and new cells take their place. Sometimes, this technique goes incorrect. New cells form when your body doesn't need them, and old or broken cells don't pass away as they ought to. The accumulation of extra cells often forms scores of tissues called a rise or tumor. Main brain tumors can be harmless or malignant.

Benign brain tumors do not contain cancer cells.

Usually, benign tumors can be removed, plus they seldom grow back again.

Benign brain tumors will often have an apparent border or edge. Cells from harmless tumors hardly ever invade cells around them. They don't really spread to other areas of your body. However, harmless tumors can press on delicate areas of the mind and cause serious health issues.

Unlike benign tumors generally in most other areas of

your body, benign brain tumors are occasionally life threatening.

Benign brain tumors could become malignant.

Malignant brain tumors (also known as brain cancer) contain cancer cells:

Malignant brain tumors are usually more serious and frequently are a threat to life.

They will probably grow rapidly and crowd or invade the close by healthy brain tissue.

Malignancy cells may break from malignant brain tumors and pass on to other areas of the mind or even to the spinal-cord.

They rarely spread to other areas of your body.

Tumor Grade

Doctors group brain tumors by grade. The standard of a tumor identifies what sort of cells look under a microscope:

Grade I: The cells is benign. The cells look almost like normal brain cells, plus they grow slowly.

Grade II: The tissues is malignant. The cells look less like normal cells than do the cells in a Grade I tumor.

Grade III: The malignant cells has cells that look completely different from normal cells. The irregular cells are positively growing (anaplastic).

Grade IV: The malignant tissues has cells that look most unusual and have a tendency to grow quickly.

Cells from low-grade tumors (marks I and II) look more normal and generally grow more gradually than cells from high-grade tumors (levels III and IV).

As time passes, a low-grade tumor could become a high-grade tumor. However, the change to a high-grade tumor happens more regularly among adults than children.

Types of Major Brain Tumors

There are various kinds of primary brain tumors. For adults, the most typical brain tumor types are astrocytoma, oligodendroglioma and meningioma.

Principal brain tumors are named based on the kind of cells or the area of the brain where they begin. For instance, most main brain tumors start in glial cells. This sort of tumor is named a glioma.

- Glioma: Gliomas start from glial cells within the supportive cells of the mind. There are many types of gliomas, classified by where they are located, and where in fact the tumor starts. Listed below are gliomas:

- Astrocytoma: The tumor comes from star-shaped glial cells called astrocytes. It could be any grade. In adults, an astrocytoma frequently occurs in the cerebrum.

- Grade I or II astrocytoma: It might be called a low-grade glioma.

- Grade III astrocytoma: It's sometimes called a high-grade or an anaplastic astrocytoma.

- Grade IV astrocytoma: It might be called a glioblastoma (GBM) or malignant astrocytic glioma.

- Oligodendroglioma: The tumor comes from cells that produce the fatty material that addresses and shields nerves. It usually occurs in the cerebrum. It's most common in middle-aged adults. It could be grade II or III.

- Meningioma: Meningiomas are usually slow-growing, benign tumors which come from the outer coverings of the mind slightly below the skull. This sort of tumor makes up about 1 / 3 of brain tumors in adults. The tumor comes up in the meninges. It could be grade I, II, or III. It is almost always benign (grade I) and expands slowly.

Among children, the most typical tumor types are:

- Medulloblastoma: The tumor usually arises in the cerebellum. It's sometimes called a primitive neuroectodermal tumor. It really is grade IV.

- Grade I or II astrocytoma: In children, this low-grade tumor occurs any place in the brain. The most frequent astrocytoma among children is juvenile pilocytic astrocytoma. It's grade I.

- Ependymoma: The tumor comes from cells that collects the ventricles or the central canal of the spinal-cord. It's mostly within children and adults. It could be grade I, II, or III.

- Brainstem glioma: The tumor occurs in the cheapest area of the brain. It's rather a low-grade or high-grade tumor. The most frequent type is diffuse intrinsic pontine glioma.

Brain Tumor: Levels and Prognostic Factors

A staging system is utilized for most other styles of

tumors in other areas of your body, to describe in which a tumor is situated, if or where they have spread, and whether it's affecting other areas of your body. However, there is absolutely no suggested systemic staging system for adult brain tumors because most major tumors do not usually pass on beyond the central anxious system. The grading system explained below is always used instead because the precise top features of a brain tumor regulate how cancerous it is and exactly how likely it is to develop.

Prognostic factors

To select the best treatment for a brain tumor, both type and grade of the tumor must be determined. There are many factors that help doctors determine the correct brain tumor treatment solution and a patient's prognosis:

> Tumor histology. As layed out in the Analysis section, an example of the tumor is removed for evaluation. Tumor histology includes the kind of tumor, the grade, and extra molecular features that

forecast how quickly the tumor can develop. Collectively, these factors can help your doctor know how the tumor will behave. These factors also may help determine a patient's treatment plans.

Grade describes certain features in the tumor that are associated with specific results. For instance, doctors may consider if the tumor cells are growing uncontrollable or if there are a great number of deceased cells. Tumors with features generally associated with growing quicker are given an increased grade. For some tumors, the low the grade, the better the prognosis.

Designed for glial tumors, the grade depends upon its features, as seen under a microscope, based on the following criteria:

- Grade I. These tumors are gradual growing and improbable to spread. They are able to often be healed with surgery.

- Grade II. These tumors are less inclined to grow and pass on but will keep coming back after treatment.

- Grade III. These tumors will have quickly dividing cells but no lifeless cells. They are able to grow quickly.

- Grade IV. Inside a grade IV tumor, cells in the tumor are positively dividing. Furthermore, the tumor has bloodstream vessel development and regions of dead tissues. These tumors can develop and pass on quickly.

Age group. In adults, a person's age group and his / her level of working, called functional position (see below) when diagnosed is among the best ways to predict a patient's prognosis. Generally, a younger adult has a much better prognosis.

Symptoms. The symptoms an individual has and exactly how long they last also may help determine prognosis. For instance, seizures and having symptoms for a long period are associated with a much better prognosis.

Degree of tumor residual. Resection is surgery to eliminate a tumor. Residual identifies how a lot of the tumor remains in the torso after surgery. A patient's prognosis is way better when every one of the tumor can be surgically removed. You can find 4 classifications:

- Gross total: The complete tumor was removed. However, microscopic cells may stay.

- Subtotal: Large servings of the tumor were removed.

- Partial: Only area of the tumor was removed.

- Biopsy only: Only a little part, used for a biopsy, was removed.

Tumor location. A tumor can develop in any area of the brain. Some tumor locations cause more harm than others, plus some tumors are harder to take care of for their location.

Molecular features. Certain hereditary mutations within the tumor can help determine prognosis. Included in these are: IDH1, IDH2, MGMT, and a 1p/19q co-deletion. Sometimes, whether a tumor has these mutations determines the kind of brain tumor that is diagnosed.

Functional neurologic status. The physician will test how well an individual can function and perform everyday activities by utilizing a practical assessment scale, like the Karnofsky Performance Scale (KPS), outlined below. An increased score indicates a much better functional status. Typically, a person who is better in a position to walk and look after themselves has a much better prognosis.

100 Normal, no complaints, no proof disease

90 In a position to keep on normal activity; small symptoms of disease

80 Normal activity with work; some symptoms of disease

70 Cares for personal; unable to keep on normal activity or energetic work

60 Requires occasional assistance but can look after needs

50 Requires considerable assistance and frequent health care

40 Disabled: requires special care and assistance

30 Severely disabled; hospitalization is indicated, but loss of life not imminent

20 Very ill, hospitalization necessary; energetic treatment necessary

10 Moribund, fatal functions progressing rainy Metastatic distributed.

A tumor that begins in the mind or spinal-cord, if cancerous, seldom spreads to other areas of your body in adults, but may grow within the CNS. Because of this, with few exceptions, tests taking a look at the other organs of your body are typically unnecessary. A tumor that does spread to other areas of the mind or spinal-cord is associated with a poorer prognosis.

Repeated tumor. A repeated tumor is one which has keep coming back after treatment. If the tumor will return, you will see another circular of checks to find out about the level of the recurrence. These testing and scans tend to be much like those done during the original analysis.

Presently, the factors in the above list will be the best indicators of the patient's prognosis. As talked about in Diagnosis, experts are looking for biomarkers in the tumor cells that will make a brain tumor simpler to diagnose and invite for the staging of a grown-up brain tumor in the foreseeable future. Researchers are also taking a look at other genetic tests that may predict a patient's prognosis. These tools may someday help doctors predict the opportunity a brain tumor will grow, develop far better treatments, and more accurately predict prognosis.

chapter 8

Where Brain Malignancies Start and Spread

A brain tumor is scores of cells in the human brain that aren't normal. A couple of two general sets of brain tumors:

- Main brain tumors begin in brain tissues and have a tendency to stay there.

- Supplementary brain tumors are more prevalent. These malignancies start someplace else in the torso and happen to be the mind. Lung, breasts, kidney, digestive tract, and skin malignancies are among the most typical malignancies that can pass on to the mind.

Some brain tumors contain malignancy cells as well as others don't:

- Benign brain tumors don't possess cancer cells.

They develop slowly, can frequently be removed, and hardly ever spread to the mind cells around them. They are able to cause problems if indeed they press on certain specific areas of the mind, though. Based on where they may be located in the mind, they could be life-threatening.

- Malignant brain tumors have cancer cells. The rates of development vary, but cells can invade healthy brain tissues close by. Malignant tumors seldom spread beyond the mind or spinal-cord.

- Marks of Brain Tumors

Tumors are graded by how normal or abnormal the cells look. Your physician use this measurement to help plan your treatment. The grading also gives you a concept of how fast the tumor may grow and spread.

Grade 1. The cells look almost normal and develop slowly. Long-term success is likely.

Grade 2. The cells look somewhat abnormal and develop gradually. The tumor may pass on to close by tissue and can recur later, maybe at a far more life-threatening grade.

Grade 3. The cells look irregular and are positively growing into close by brain cells. These tumors have a tendency to recur.

Grade 4. The cells look most unusual and develop and spread quickly.

Some tumors change. Hardly ever some harmless tumors can change malignant, and a lower-grade tumor may come back at an increased grade.

Types of Brain Tumors

In adults, the most typical types of brain cancer are:

- Astrocytomas. These usually occur in the biggest area of the brain, the cerebrum. They could be any grade. They often times cause seizures or changes in behavior.

- Meningiomas . They are the most typical principal brain tumors in adults. They are likely that occurs in your 70s or 80s. They arise in the meninges, the liner of the mind. They could be grade 1, 2, or 3.

They are generally harmless and grow gradually.

- Oligodendrogliomas. These occur in the cells that produce the covering that protects nerves. They're usually grade 1, 2, or 3. They often grow slowly and do not spread to close by tissue.

How Brain Tumor Is Treated

Your treatment depends on the sort and grade of the tumor, where it's located, its size, as well as your age group and health.

Surgery is usually the first treatment. For grade 1 tumors, it might be enough. It's possible that the cancers can be removed. But even if it isn't, the surgery can decrease the size and relieve symptoms.

Radiation therapy can be used after surgery to get rid of any tumor cells that stay in the region. If surgery isn't a choice, you might have only rays therapy.

Chemotherapy may also be used to wipe out brain

malignancy cells. It really is given by mouth area, IV, or, less often, in wafers a doctor puts in the mind.

Targeted therapy may be used to treat certain types of brain tumors. These drugs assault specific elements of tumor cells and avoid tumors from growing and distributing.

Your doctor could also recommend combined therapies.

chapter 9

WHAT'S Glioblastoma?

Glioblastoma is a kind of brain cancers. It's the most typical kind of malignant brain tumor among adults. Which is usually very intense, this means it can develop fast and spread quickly.

Although there is absolutely no cure, there are treatments to help ease symptoms.

Where It Forms in the mind

Glioblastoma is a kind of astrocytoma, a malignancy that forms from star-shaped cells in the mind called astrocytes. In adults, this malignancy usually begins in the cerebrum, the biggest part of the human brain.

Glioblastoma tumors make their own blood circulation, which helps them grow. It's possible for these to invade normal brain tissues.

How Common COULD IT BE?

Brain malignancies aren't common. So when they happen, about 4 out of 5 aren't glioblastomas. Men will have them than women. And chances rise with age group. Doctors diagnose about 14,000 glioblastoma instances in the U.S. every year.

Symptoms

Because glioblastomas grow quickly, strain on the brain usually causes the first symptoms. Based on where in fact the tumor is, it can cause:

- Constant headaches.

- Seizures.

- Vomiting.

- Trouble thinking.

- Changes in feeling or personality.

- Double or blurry vision.

- Trouble speaking

Diagnosis

A neurologist (a health care provider who specializes in diagnosing and treating brain disorders) will provide you with an entire exam. You can find an MRI or CT scan and other exams, depending on your symptoms.

Treatment

The purpose of glioblastoma treatment is to slow and control tumor growth and help your home as comfortably as you possibly can. You will find four treatments, and many people get several type:

- Surgery is the first treatment. The doctor tries to eliminate as a lot of the tumor as you can. In high-risk regions of the mind, it might not be possible to eliminate everything.

- Radiation is utilized to kill as much leftover tumor

cells as is possible after surgery. Additionally, it may slow the development of tumors that can not be removed by surgery.

- Chemotherapy also may help. Temozolomide is the most typical chemotherapy medication doctors use for glioblastoma. Chemo can cause short-term part results, but it's significantly less harmful than it used to be.

Doctors can treat glioblastoma that comes home with another chemotherapy medication called carmustine (or BCNU).

Electric field therapy uses electric fields to focus on cells in the tumor without hurting normal cells. To get this done, doctors put electrodes on the head. The device is named Optune. You obtain it with chemotherapy after surgery and rays. The FDA has approved it for both recently diagnosed people and folks whose glioblastoma keeps coming back.

At major cancer centers, you may even be capable of geting experimental treatments or dental chemotherapy, that you take at home.

These treatments can help with symptoms and perhaps put the tumor into remission in a few people. In remission, symptoms may let up or vanish for a while.

Glioblastomas often regrow. If that occurs, doctors might be able to address it with surgery and a different form of rays and chemotherapy.

Palliative care is also very important to anyone with a significant illness. It offers caring for your pain and the feelings you might be working with, and also other symptoms from your cancers. The target is to enhance the grade you will ever have.

You may even want to ask your physician if there's a

clinical trial that might be a good fit for you.

Outlook and Success Rates

Many things make a difference how well someone does when they have cancer, including glioblastomas. Doctors often can't anticipate what someone's life span will be if indeed they have a glioblastoma. However they do have figures that track what size groups of individuals who've experienced these conditions have a tendency to do as time passes.

For glioblastoma, the success rates are:

Twelve months: 40.2%

2 yrs: 17.4%

Five years: 5.6%

These numbers can't predict exactly what will happen to a person, though. A person's age group, kind of tumor, and general health are likely involved. As treatments improve, people recently identified as having these intense brain tumors may have a much better outcome.

what does grade 4 astrocytoma mean?

Glioblastomas are occasionally called grade 4 astrocytoma tumors. Tumors are graded on the level from 1 to 4 structured about how different they look from normal cells. The grade shows how fast the tumor will probably develop and spread.

A grade 4 tumor is the most aggressive and fastest-growing type. It could spread during your brain rapidly.

Types of glioblastoma

You can find two types of glioblastoma:

- Major (de novo) is the most typical kind of glioblastoma. It's also the most intense form.

- Supplementary glioblastoma is less common and slower growing. It usually begins from a lower-grade, less intense astrocytoma. Supplementary glioblastoma impacts about ten percent of individuals with this kind of brain malignancy. A lot of people who understand this form of malignancy are age group 45 or more youthful.

Glioblastomas often grow in the frontal and temporal lobes of the mind. They may also be found in the mind stem, cerebellum, other areas of the mind, and the spinal-cord.

Survival rates and life span

The median survival time with glioblastoma is 15 to 16 months Trusted Source in people who get surgery, chemotherapy, and rays treatment. Median means fifty percent of most patients with this tumor survive to the amount of time.

Everyone with glioblastoma differs. Some individuals don't survive for as long. Other people can survive up to five years or even more, although it's uncommon.

In children

Children with higher-grade tumors have a tendency to survive much longer than adults. About twenty five percent of kids who've this tumor live for five years or even more.

Extending life span

New treatments are extending life span even more. People whose tumors have a good hereditary marker called MGMT methylation have better success rates.

MGMT is a gene that maintenance damaged cells. When chemotherapy kills glioblastoma cells, MGMT fixes them. MGMT methylation helps prevent this repair and means that more tumor cells are wiped out.

Glioblastoma treatments

Glioblastoma can be hard to take care of. It increases quickly, and they have finger-like projections in to the normal brain that are hard to eliminate with surgery. These tumors also contain many types of cells. Some treatments may work very well on some cells, however, not on others.

Treatment for glioblastoma usually involves:

- surgery to eliminate as a lot of the tumor as it can be.

- radiation to get rid of any tumor cells which were left out after surgery

- chemotherapy with the medication temozolomide (Temodar)

Other drugs which may be used to take care of this cancers include:

bevacizumab (Avastin)

polifeprosan 20 with carmustine implant (Gliadel)

lomustine (Ceenu)

New treatments for glioblastoma are being analyzed in clinical tests. These treatments include:

- immunotherapy - making use of your body's disease fighting capability to kill cancers cells.

- gene therapy - mending defective genes to take care of cancer.

- stem cell therapy - using early cells called stem cells to take care of cancer.

- vaccine therapy - conditioning your body's disease fighting capability to battle off cancer.

- individualized medicine - also known as targeted therapy

If these and other treatments are approved, they could 1

day enhance the outlook for individuals with glioblastoma.

Causes and risk factors

Doctors don't know very well what causes glioblastoma. Like other malignancies, it begins when cells start to develop uncontrollably and form tumors. This cell development may have something regarding gene changes.

You're much more likely to understand this kind of tumor if you're:

male

over age group 50

of Caucasian or Asian heritage

Glioblastoma symptoms

Glioblastoma causes symptoms when it presses on elements of the human brain. If the tumor isn't large, you will possibly not have any observeable symptoms. Which symptoms you have depends upon where in the human brain the tumor is situated.

Symptoms range from:

- headaches.

- nausea and vomiting.

- Sleepiness.

- weakness using one aspect of the body.

- memory loss.

- problems with talk and language.

- personality and disposition changes.

- muscle weakness.

- dual vision or blurry vision.

- lack of appetite.

- seizures

Acknowledgments

The Glory of this book success goes to God Almighty and my beautiful Family, Fans, Readers & well-wishers, Customers and Friends for their endless support and encouragements.

www.ingramcontent.com/pod-product-compliance
Lightning Source LLC
Chambersburg PA
CBHW020301030426
42336CB00010B/849